The Complete Manual

of

NATURAL ALLERGY CONTROL

Written and Researched by

DR. DAVID G. WILLIAMS

ISBN 0944649-00-9

Dedicated to my many valued patients, friends and family who have suffered a variety of allergy problems. Their relentless search for relief became my inspiration for compiling the research for this book.

First Edition, 1987
Second Edition, 1990
Third Edition, 1993

Copyright 1987
Mountain Home Publishing

CONTENTS

CHAPTER 8

CHAPTER 9

CHAPTER 10

INTRODUCTION

ALLERGIES...Minor Inconvenience or Growing Threat?

Allergies are rapidly becoming one of the most common problems in our world today. The Allergy Foundation of America states that "...allergies may constitute one of the most widespread, undiagnosed diseases in the United States". It has been estimated that at least one-fourth of the population of the United States have severe allergy problems and probably 50% experience the so-called minor allergic ailments. Exact figures on the full extent of the problem remains a mystery since thousands of sufferers try to handle the problem on their own with over-the-counter medications, diet restrictions or avoiding exposure to pollen-laden areas. School age children are some of the worst victims. Over one-third of all chronic diseases in children under the age of 18 are caused by hay fever, asthma and other allergies!

Allergies can be more than just a periodic inconvenience. Asthma alone causes thousands of deaths each year. Deaths from emphysema, another chronic respiratory condition involving the degeneration of the alveolar walls in the lungs, are increasing at an almost unbelievable rate each year. Allergies to foods, molds, cigarette smoke, various

1

chemicals and airborne particles are now suspected to be some of the underlying causes of many disease processes such as: arthritis, cardiovascular disease and some cancers.

The dollar cost to allergy sufferers runs into the hundreds of millions. It is estimated that over $500 million is spent on injections and medicines alone. Millions more are spent on various sensitivity tests, many of which give questionable or inconsistent results. The greatest costs borne by the allergic individual have very little to do with money.

Current treatment regimes virtually turn the allergy sufferer into a prisoner in their own home. The joys of participating in outdoor activities are lost. Allergic children are forced to forego the exploration of the great outdoors and the educational comradery of those their own age. Restrictive diets to avoid any possible allergic reaction can cause additional stress and imbalance to an already weakened immune system. In short, if you are one of the millions of allergy sufferers in this country you have most likely lost many of the personal freedoms associated with good health.

The problems with allergies are not new. As far back as 3000 B.C. records indicate that Shen Nung, the Emperor of China, noted that certain foods caused skin ulcerations in pregnant women. The dietary restrictions in the Old Testament are thought to be based on allergic complications. The early Greek physicians made numerous references to allergy problems. Hippocrates wrote, "It is a bad thing to give milk to persons having headache". Lucretius in the first century B. C. uttered the famous phrase, "one mans meat is another mans poison". Allergies have been around for thousands of years. After you get a clear understanding of just exactly what an allergy really is, and the current "high tech" diagnostic tests and treatment programs, you'll see why allergies will still be around for thousands of years to come.

CHAPTER 1

THE CAUSE OF AN ALLERGY IS CLOSER THAN YOU THINK!

If you understand just exactly what an allergy is, you will be in a much better position to make an informed choice about the various methods of treatment.

An allergy is an abnormal physiological reaction to a specific substance that is normally harmless to others.

The white blood cells in your body protect you from harmful substances like bacteria and viruses, known as antigens. They do this by producing proteins known as antibodies. In the allergic individual the immune system becomes confused and produces antibodies against harmless substances like pollens, molds, dust or foods. These antibodies travel by way of the blood stream to all parts of the body. When they reach their destination, usually an area containing mucus deposits, they attach to mast cells. The next time one of the allergens enter the bloodstream from the digestive system, the lungs, the skin or even by injection, the sensitized mast cell releases a substance called histamine.

Histamine and histamine-related substances cause the typical allergic reactions...inflammation, swelling and smooth muscle contractions. In the case of asthma, the smooth circular muscles of the bronchial tubes constrict. In hives the swelling and inflammation of the skin occurs, or in hay fever the blood vessels dilate or enlarge in the nasal passages. Allergic reactions can cause a congested or runny nose, itching, breathing difficulties, sneezing, skin wheals, or even more serious complaints like headaches, diarrhea, nausea and even death.

What is considered an antigen in the healthy person could be an allergen to the allergic individual. Remember Lucretius' statement that "one mans meat is another mans poison"? Regardless of what you may have been told, keep in mind that the allergen (pollen, dust, mold, food, etc.) is not the culprit. It is the exact same substance that exists in harmony with most people. The real problem is how your body reacts to it. An allergic reaction indicates that your body is out of balance with nature. Let's now take a brief look at how the current allergy treatments completely avoid this basic principle.

You can spend literally thousands of dollars on elaborate testing to determine what specific substances "you are allergic to". The substances are then treated as the problem. Accordingly, the allergen must then be avoided at all costs. Changing occupations or even moving to a different part of the country are not uncommon recommendations. Completely eliminating hundreds of different foods from the diet is also not unheard of. Entire volumes have been written to assist you in detecting and avoiding certain foods or products. Any one of these volumes can practically turn the average citizen into a full-time detective. Also, we can't forget the steroid-type drugs that round out these treatment programs. In an effort to ease the symptoms of an allergic response, drugs that suppress the entire immune system are readily available.

Other treatment programs involve desensitization injections. Gradually increased, minute dosages of the allergens are injected into the body. Desensitization usually offers some temporary relief and has been shown to be about 20% to 25% effective in treating all types of allergies. Rarely are any food allergies permanently cured with this method. The treatment costs are very expensive (between $1,500 and $2,500) and may last for years.

Even if these approaches were less expensive or got better results, the underlying cause of the allergy has not been addressed. Again, the allergen is not the problem. If it was, everyone exposed to it would develop an allergic reaction. The allergen is not abnormal, the response generated by the immune system is abnormal.

CHAPTER 2

CURRENT MEDICAL ALLERGY TREATMENTS...HIGH-TECH COMBINED WITH LOW SENSE?

OVER-THE-COUNTER MEDICATION

Over-the-counter medication is probably the most common form of allergy treatment and no doubt the most lucrative from the drug manufacturer's point of view. In private, representatives of the drug industry readily admit that drugs used to <u>treat</u> a condition are vastly more profitable than those drugs which eliminate it. Allergy medications are "a dream come true". Without exception, the medications do nothing more than suppress the symptoms associated with allergies while doing absolutely nothing in the way of eliminating the problem. A prime example of this is nasal sprays.

Sales of over-the-counter nasal sprays are now about $150 million a year. Although sales continue to climb, very few of the users realize the dangers of long term usage. Most sprays contain a drug that mimics the actions of a hormone produced naturally by the adrenal glands. It causes the small blood vessels in the nose to constrict. If the spray is used steadily for five to seven days the user experiences the so-called "rebound phenomenon". This is a cycle of discomfort, short relief and then more discomfort. (Sounds like a description of a drug addiction doesn't it?)

With repeated use, the small muscles that constrict the blood vessels eventually fatigue. This in turn, allows the blood vessels to expand which causes the congestion to return. It then takes even larger doses to shrink the vessels and reopen the nose. Once you get caught up in this cycle, trying to unblock a stuffy nose with nasal sprays, it's much like trying to put out a fire by throwing gasoline on it. Continued use leads to sinus infections and chronic congestion as well as more serious problems like visual disturbances and added stress to the immune system, especially to the adrenal glands.

Drugs interfere with the body's natural healing processes which is a questionable tactic for dealing with allergies. An example to look at would be the runny nose. This discharge is the body's method of getting rid of the excess mucus. The coughing and sneezing only enhances the process. A cold is how the body cleans the airways of trapped debris and mucus. To illustrate this further, consider the cigarette smoker.

Toxins, debris and mucus accumulate in the lungs of a smoker much faster than in a non-smoker. In fact, the body of a heavy smoker must go through a temporary survival cleaning everyday. The early morning ritual of hacking, coughing and spitting up phlegm can be equated with having a constant cold. Although no one in their right mind would recommend that a smoker should suppress this discharge, it has become the standard procedure to suppress any elimination during the "common cold". Millions of dollars worth of drugs are prescribed and purchased over-the-counter each year to suppress the elimination of mucus during a cold or flu.

PRESCRIPTION DRUGS

Prescription drugs are another common approach to allergy control. The most common of the hundreds of allergy drugs are the antihistamines and the cortisone derivatives.

Antihistamines may help alleviate some allergy symptoms, but they have to be taken constantly. Their side effects are many. "Thickening of the bronchial secretions" is one of the most common. Making the mucus thicker keeps the body from being able to get rid of it. What starts out as a simple head or chest cold can gradually turn into a full blown case of pneumonia. Other side effects include shock, low blood pressure, heart racing and palpitations, anemia, vision and hearing problems, nausea, vomiting, constipation and diarrhea to name just a few.

Continued use of cortisone derivatives can suppress the entire immune system Your ability to produce antibodies is diminished. Not producing antibodies for pollen or molds may help relieve some allergy symptoms; however, not being able to produce any antibodies can leave you defenseless against more serious degenerative diseases. Besides depleting your adrenal glands, other side-effects involve:

A Potassium-Sodium imbalance
(leading to water retention)

Swelling and High Blood Pressure

Ulcers

Heart Problems

Inability To Heal

The use of drugs may be a high price to pay for relief of a stuffy nose and watery eyes.

DESENSITIZATION THERAPY

Desensitization therapy involves the injection of increasing amounts of allergens in a salt solution into the bloodstream. Usually the patient can expect only temporary relief at best and the process may take as long as 6 months to 2 years to achieve results.

Even though this therapy has just become popular in the last few years, it was started over seventy-five years ago by a Dr. Leonard Noon in Britain. A simplified explanation of how it works may help you understand why injecting the same antigen that causes problems can be expected to bring relief.

Apparently, steady doses (usually 1 to 2 weeks) of the antigens deplete the allergic antibodies. When the antibodies are depleted you no longer have a reaction to that substance. On the down side, since your body is constantly producing antibodies and since this therapy works best on dust, molds, pollens, etc., you may be taking injections indefinitely. The frequency would depend on what substances you're allergic to and what seasons they occur in.

Generally, this type of therapy has no effect on food or chemical allergies. In part, this is because food allergies as you'll see later, often involve an underlying digestive imbalance.

ISOLATION FROM THE ALLERGEN

Isolation from the allergen is another accepted approach. If you are allergic to a particular area, you may be asked to move. Many people have changed occupations, broken social and family ties and relocated, only to discover that the new area is loaded with new and different allergens. The isolation approach seems to be the ultimate in trying to run away from the environment, rather than balancing the immune system so the body can co-exist in harmony. Even if it was possible to place the allergic sufferer in a completely sterile environment this would not correct the real problem....the body's abnormal reaction to a normally harmless substance.

ELIMINATION DIETS

Elimination diets are an approach to the allergy solution that has launched volumes of books and turned thousands into nutritional experts overnight. Some health practitioners, nutritionists and "clinical ecologists" focus on certain foods as being the allergens. The treatment regime consists of eliminating the offending food item from the diet. Unfortunately, the list of foods involved is usually quite long. The most common items eliminated are sugar, milk, eggs, chocolate, wheat, corn, beans, nuts, soft drinks and various fruits. If eliminating the foods on this list doesn't seem like it would be a problem, just read a few labels. Almost every product in the grocery store will contain either sugar, milk, eggs or corn extract.

The offending foods are determined by the "elimination diet", and *Dr. Author Coca's pulse test. (*Complete instructions for this screening self-test are outlined in Chapter 6.)

One of the positive aspects of this program is the constant awareness of what foods are being eaten. Also, emphasis placed on unprocessed, unadulterated foods and nutritional supplements is a positive and welcome trend.

Unfortunately, with this program, many people never "recover" from certain foods and their permanent diet lacks some of the most wholesome and rejuvenating grains, fruits and vegetables placed on this planet for our use. Again, the idea that the allergen (food) is the cause of the allergy shows the obvious flaw in this approach.

CHAPTER 3

NATURAL APPROACHES TO ALLERGIES

First, I should clarify (or confuse) that the elimination diet and the isolation programs could probably fall somewhere under the category of natural approaches. However, both of these usually involve the use of medication and purists of the next two schools of thought, would not consider them totally natural.

MEGA-VITAMIN THERAPY

Mega-vitamin therapy attempts to address the allergy problem two ways.

First, in large doses, certain vitamins have a drug-like effect on the body. Without the side-effects they can alter the body's chemical balance. For example, prolonged use of large niacin doses (several grams a day) can elevate blood sugar levels. Large doses of vitamin K can influence blood clotting factors. In allergies, large doses of vitamin C (to "acidify the system") and B vitamins are common recommendations. In larger dosages, the vitamin C complex, vitamin E, fish oil and Evening Primrose oil all have anti-inflammatory capabilities. Their actions are somewhat similar to cortisone, aspirin and many arthritis drugs. (By blocking the formation of arachadonic acid into prostaglandins they limit inflammation with only minimal side-effects.)

Secondly, mega-vitamin therapy works to eliminate the deficiencies common in allergy sufferers, most commonly the B vitamins and vitamin C. Extra stress, as you'll see later, depletes these important nutrients.

Mega-vitamin therapy is a very useful tool and remarkable results have been obtained using it, but it should be considered just that...a tool. It is only one method to help in balancing the immune system and enabling it to respond normally to the environment.

HOMEOPATHY, BEE POLLEN, HONEY AND HONEYCOMB

Homeopathy, bee pollen, honey and honeycomb can be excellent natural remedies for allergy problems, but again, don't address the root of the problem.

Homeopathy is a branch of the "like cures like" theory. Solutions that contain very minute amounts of the offending allergen are introduced into the body either orally or by injection. Oral homeopathic remedies for various conditions can be purchased at most health food stores. Originally, it is reported that homeopaths used around eighty different ingredients. Today, there are several thousand plants and chemicals comprising the practice.

Bee pollen, honey and honeycomb, basically work on the same principle. Each of these contain small amounts of pollen from the local flowering trees, bushes, plants, vegetables, etc. By consuming these in the raw form, many allergics have become naturally desensitized. As far as I can tell, no actual controlled research has been conducted on the use of honey or bee pollen; however, I have personally seen very favorable results in patients using a teaspoon daily of local raw honey. (Note: Some authorities urge extreme caution in the use of bee pollen which itself can cause severe allergic reactions. Honey and honeycomb seem to be of less concern.)

These products have the same underlying flaw as desensitization injections; however, they may be much easier to take from both a financial and pain standpoint.

CHAPTER 4

WHAT'S MISSING?

All of the therapies (medical and natural) fail to fully address the abnormal response of the immune system. Vitamin therapy comes closest to the right direction, but only when it is used specifically to help rebuild the immune system and not as a drug substitute. Many people feel comfortable trading their allergies for a handful of daily vitamins. I have nothing against taking vitamins and take several myself, but when the body is in balance with its environment, you should be able to take vitamins only for maintenance and preventative purposes. If you <u>have to</u> take vitamins everyday to constantly suppress an allergy problem, your immune and/or digestive system needs help.

If the basic cause of allergies was truly the environment (pollen, dust, molds, cat fur, lint, food, etc.), everyone would have allergies. Someone might argue that everyone is allergic to certain chemicals such as DDT or gasoline, but you must remember these are not allergens. An allergen is a substance that triggers an allergic response to the sufferer, but is normally harmless to others. We're not allergic to DDT, gasoline, various food additives, etc., they are poisons. They're poisonous to all living creatures. No human can build up an immunity to drinking gasoline.

Another major stumbling block to getting rid of allergies is the dualistic philosophy of good and evil. Man who is good is constantly at war with his hostile environment. Each day our bodies are attacked by millions of life-threatening organisms. Everyday we struggle to cope with the cruelties and harshness of mother nature. Germs and microbes are viewed as enemies posing a threat to our very existence. Drugs become our weapons to seek out and destroy these enemies. As enemies (bacteria, viruses, etc.) mutate to survive, drugs that lose their effectiveness must be replaced with stronger more virile ones.

We see this same theme repeated daily on television commercials and documentaries. It is taught in our elementary and medical school biology classes. Mans fight for survival has become so entrenched into our thinking it's difficult to even picture man in harmony with the environment.

Man was created to exist in harmony with Earth and all its splendor. Microbes and bacteria are essential to our survival. Our intestines harbor colonies of friendly bacteria. They are essential for proper digestion and the absorption of nutrients. Bacteria and the so-called germs are on practically every surface we touch. They are part of the natural chain of life on Earth and they're here to stay...thank goodness, since we couldn't live without them.

Allergens are now viewed in the same light as germs. A menace to man that must either be avoided or eliminated. The fallacy of this way of thinking should be obvious when you consider that every substance is a possible allergen. If you've been reading some of the popular health magazines lately, you may have seen reports that some people have been found to be allergic to exercise, heat or cold. I have seen hundreds of allergy test profiles showing patients are allergic to almost everything in the environment. Some unfortunate souls have literally been subjected to bread and water diets. (If they can locate the proper type of bread.)

Even with the gross inconsistency and questionable value of allergy testing, thousands subject themselves to it each year. The fact that every substance on the face of the Earth has the capability of triggering an allergy attack in someone, hasn't seemed to discourage the relentless allergists. They feel it's their ordained duty to subject the confused patient to everything from cat fur to corn syrup in search of the wicked allergen.

The allergy sufferer seems to be caught in the middle of all of this. Seeking relief, he has been everywhere. First, trying over-the-counter preparations and home remedies recommended by well-meaning friends and relatives. Finding no relief, he visits the family medical doctor who prescribes various antihistamines and cortisone medications. After only temporary relief, he is referred to an allergy specialist who uses the latest in testing and desensitizing procedures. After months of sporadic relief the decision is made to try the natural route. Nutritionists tell him the allergies are due to vitamin and mineral deficiencies. Hundreds of pills and dollars later his medical doctor learns he wants to try natural methods. He is then referred to a psychologist who uses bio-feedback and other behavior modification techniques. Further searching leads to a doctor of chiropractic who offers to correct spinal nerve interference and the lowered resistance it causes. Later, an acupuncturist, an herbalist and a homeopathic physician all become involved in the endless cycle.

The allergic patient does get varying amounts of relief and truly feels every health practitioner has something to offer; however, as time passes, the allergies always return and the patient is confused. At this point several things can occur.

The patient may re-enter the cycle hoping some new technique or treatment procedure has been developed. He may look for a new doctor or new herbalist, etc., hoping their background and training may hold the key. Oftentimes, in depressed and weakened state, the patient decides to live with the problem. In the back of his mind he can't help but wonder if it's his fate to suffer with this problem or if he has some mental disturbance that encourages this condition.

Regardless of what you've been lead to believe or might like to believe...there is no quick cure for allergies. Only your body can cure. No drug, vitamin therapy or doctor can cure. However, any or all of these may be needed to assist the body in performing its miracles.

The ultimate miracle of healing is present in your body. The body is constantly working to maintain balance and harmony with its environment.

Everything in our environment affects our health. Light and sound waves, electromagnetic energy, the air we breath, the thoughts we think, the water we drink and the food we eat, all influence our state of health. Our most basic tie with the environment involves our daily intake of food and drink. As you'll see, this important link with the outside world influences our health even before we are born.

CHAPTER 5

HOW DO ALLERGIES GET STARTED...WHERE DO THEY COME FROM?

Your susceptibility to developing allergies begins before birth. Our weaknesses and strengths are an accumulation from everyone before us. You carry genetic remnants of everyone in your ancestry. At the time of your conception, the remnants, traits, weaknesses or strengths, etc., become either expressed in your physical make-up or held dormant for expression in future generations or triggered by some event later in life.

You may have been told you inherited hay fever from your mother or that hay fever runs in your family. What many doctors describe as being inherited is actually just a weakness or susceptibility to developing hay fever. Everyone has the proverbial "weak link". It's to your benefit to determine your weak link so you can adjust your lifestyle and living habits to avoid problems in the weak organs or body systems. Look for patterns of disease and cause of deaths in the current and past generations of your family. By all means, use your doctor as a source of information. He or she can help you evaluate your areas of weakness as we give you lifestyle guidelines tailored to your particular needs. As Dr. Roger Williams explained it, you have "biochemical individuality". This accounts for the fact that no one vitamin, drug or therapy will always work for everyone with the same condition.

By knowing your weaknesses you can adjust your diet, vitamin intake and exercise program to help you live a healthier and longer life. Many allergy sufferers inherit a weak digestive system. An inability to produce sufficient hydrochloric acid or digestive enzymes is a common finding. In these cases, correcting the allergy problem may be as simple as adding enzyme supplements to the diet.

Your weaknesses, strengths and overall health was greatly influenced by your mother's diet before birth. The fetus is highly susceptible to toxins, radiation, even ultrasound waves, etc., especially during the first three months of development. It is during this period that the actual formation and development of the glands and organs occur. The fetus receives all of its nourishment and support from the mother by way of the placenta. Nutrients and even certain antibodies are passed to the child. What the mother eats and drinks can have profound effects on the overall strength and development of the newborn. Fetal development can be divided into four distinct areas.

1. The first 7 days...implantation of the fertilized egg.

2. The next 21 days...major body systems are formed.

3. The next 63 days...body systems begin to develop and the organs and glands now start to form.

4.   The next 189 days...development continues with overall strengthening.

When you stop to realize that the effects of aspirin, medications, alcohol, cigarette smoke, etc., can linger in the body for days, it's easy to see how the fetus can be put at risk. The lightening like speed at which cells are dividing and developing into organs and glands, especially during the first three months, make the fetus particularly vulnerable to outside influences. It is during this time that many congenital deformities (missing limbs, mental retardation, etc.) can occur. Even without an obvious defect, the newborn's weakened immune system may leave it with a "susceptibility" toward allergies in the future. Whether or not this individual actually ever develops allergies in the future may very well depend on his/her lifestyle. Additional stress to the immune system could hamper its ability to react normally to the environment (i.e. allergies). This stress can be either direct or indirect.

An example of direct stress would be the individual whose body is unable to produce a particular digestive enzyme, such as the one needed to break down the amino acid, tyramine. Without this enzyme, eating certain foods containing tyramine like chocolate, some cheeses and red wine will cause an accumulation of tyramine in the bloodstream. This buildup triggers an allergic reaction usually in the form of a migraine headache. Any foods that aren't properly digested can place direct stress on the immune system.

Indirectly, many things can weaken the immune system. Toxins from chronic constipation tend to overload the liver, spleen and lymphatic system, which are all key parts of the immune system. Too many refined carbohydrates (sugar) deplete the adrenal glands and their ability to combat stress. Psychological problems can cause an overactive parasympathetic nervous system. Nervous system degeneration and endocrine gland dysfunction can lead to abnormal sensitivity. Allergies, depression, irritability and learning disabilities are only a few of the possible results.

Allergies are a multi-faceted problem and their correction requires a multi-faceted solution. Even though the problem of allergies may be complex and complicated, the solution is quite simple. Several areas need to be considered when you decide to get rid of allergy problems. But as you'll see, anyone can make the simple adjustments necessary to regain freedom from allergies.

CHAPTER 6

SYSTEMATIC PROGRAM FOR ELIMINATING ALLERGIES

Any program designed to eliminate allergies must help the body in its job to exist in harmony with its environment. There are three stages necessary to accomplish this.

The first stage involves the breakdown and removal of accumulated waste. Everyone accumulates a certain amount of waste material. What we eat, drink and breath contributes to waste buildup in our body. The process of life itself, the constant dying and replacement of body cells, plays a major role as does lack of exercise, past use of drugs (legal or illegal), bowel habits and even our thoughts and emotions.

This first stage is referred to as detoxification. Without detoxification, no permanent results can be achieved.

The second stage involves the healing crisis. We have almost been trained into believing that a healing crisis should be avoided at all cost. Let's take a closer look at the necessity for the healing crisis.

After the house cleaning or detoxification in stage one, if your body is strong enough, it will begin to replace old cells and tissue. During this replacement process you may actually experience more symptoms than you had originally. Fever, mucus drainage, sore muscles and joints, headaches, foul smelling breath, feces and urine are just a few of the common complaints that accompany this phase of healing. This whole group of unpleasant symptoms is referred to as the "healing crisis". The more waste products you've accumulated during your lifetime or the longer you've suppressed their elimination with medications, mega-vitamins, etc., the worse the healing crisis can be. Since no two people are the same, everyone may react differently during this time. Someone who has lived on a super clean diet and exercised regularly, may pass through this stage with little or no problems in a couple of days. Others in poor health with a lifetime of the "normal American diet" may need a longer, less drastic cleansing program I'll explain later.

Stage three involves the time of rebuilding. Only after the body removes the waste and toxins it has accumulated, will it fully concentrate on repairing and rebuilding. Many allergy treatment programs skip the first two stages I've mentioned and concentrate on stage three alone. If you've ever been guilty of this (we all have, at some time or another), you end up treating just the symptoms of the allergy and not the cause, i.e. an abnormal response by your immune system. Failure to properly use the body's rebuilding ability is a serious mistake. Your body's ability to rebuild can be your strongest tool in eliminating allergies as well as other problems.

Some researchers state that every cell in the body is replaced within a seven year period. We know the body is constantly replacing old worn-out tissue with new. The outside layer of skin is shed and replaced on a continual basis. Long-time cigarette smokers show almost totally new lung tissue in a few years after kicking the habit. (Granted, without an elimination stage some residue and waste will always remain.)

The new cells being made can only be as good as the raw materials used to create them. If you've gone to the effort of detoxifying your body, you should concentrate on only ingesting the finest ingredients for your body to use as building blocks. This means natural whole foods, constructive thoughts and emotions and proper exercise to help stimulate circulation and encourage waste removal. Health must become a way of living. You earn good health and freedom from allergies.

Freedom from allergies cannot be achieved by fasting and elimination diets followed by junk food, nor by following the best diets and exercise programs accompanied by a weak elimination system. You can however, be free from allergies by restoring your immune system's ability to respond normally to its environment.

STAGES 1 AND 2: DETOXIFICATION AND THE HEALING CRISIS

Many methods are available to detoxify the body. In fact, entire books have been written on detoxifying diets, water fasts, juice fasts, etc. I will cover just a few of the methods I have found to be successful in dealing with allergies. The method you use should be determined after a discussion with your doctor. Again, no one method will be suitable for everyone.

1. FASTING

Fasting is probably the oldest and best known of the techniques used for detoxification and tissue cleansing. The traditional fast allows only water and may last from a single day to several weeks. I personally prefer a modified fast using juices as I'll explain later.

Fasting nowadays doesn't enjoy the popularity it once had. Today, fasting is looked upon as a form of protest or irrational behavior by extremists. Despite the fact that fasting has proven to be very effective, its therapeutic use has diminished. One of the reasons for its demise can be attributed to the quest for instant relief from an ailment. Very few people are willing to make any sacrifice today for rewards of better health in the future. Unfortunately, our society has come to expect immediate gratification and results.

Several biblical references are made to the use and benefits of fasting and even today, some religions advocate fasting one day a week. I feel a cleansing fast at least once a year would benefit most everyone.

I have intentionally not given a step by step plan for a strict water fast. If you intend to do such a fast, I would recommend you further research the idea by reading more on the topic in your local health library and consulting your doctor. A water fast can be a miraculous healing experience; however, you need to familiarize yourself with the proper way to break the fast, etc., in order to gain full benefit.

Many people, due to a weakened state of health, are unable to participate in a strict water fast and fortunately there are other cleansing methods available.

2. JUICE FASTING:

Juice fasting is one method I highly recommend for detoxification. Certain fresh juices can supply the body with all the elements needed during detoxification. If you are fortunate enough to own a juicer, you've probably tried fresh carrot juice. Carrot juice seems to be the best overall rejuvenation and cleansing juice. A good program involves drinking one 8 oz. glass of fresh carrot juice every 3 to 4 hours. Properly extracted juice can be digested and assimilated in a very short time. Some authorities say as fast as 15 to 30 minutes.

It is important that you properly juice the carrots and not simply blend them whole. By drinking only the juice without the pulp and fiber, you don't place a burden on the digestive organs. Your body will still be able to concentrate on waste removal instead of spending hours on digestive chores.

The length of time spent on a juice fast and the method of breaking the fast is similar to a water fast. Most experts don't recommend fasting over a week or ten days without experienced supervision.

Breaking a fast must be done properly. Most programs have a two or four day transition period before returning to a normal diet. I have outlined a typical three day transition period to give you an idea of how a fast can be broken.

1ST DAY FOLLOWING A JUICE OR WATER FAST:

In the morning, eat a small piece of fruit. Apples and pears are especially good since they contain the roughage you will gradually need to re-introduce into the diet.

For lunch, a vegetable or potato soup would be a good choice.

In the evening, a small portion of the soup or the juice (i.e. carrot) used during the fast.

2ND DAY AFTER A FAST:

In the morning, eat more fruit. In addition to apples or pears, you may select figs or prunes.

For lunch, a small fresh salad.

For dinner, soup again.

3RD DAY AFTER A FAST:

In the morning, fruit again and you may add yogurt. Wheat germ sprinkled on top makes for a nice nutty change.

For lunch a large fresh salad and even a baked or boiled potato with the skin left on. Use a small amount of butter or yogurt for topping on the potato.

For dinner, soup again.

4TH DAY AFTER A FAST:

You can now begin to incorporate clean healthy foods back into your diet. You should be able to eat normal sized portions and three meals daily. Don't go to the trouble of fasting and then return to a diet of garbage!

IMPORTANT POINTS TO REMEMBER ABOUT FASTING

Since the purpose of a fast is to cleanse and detoxify your body, don't be surprised if you experience detoxification symptoms. Nausea, fatigue, diarrhea, irritability, headaches, muscle aches, or other flu-like symptoms may accompany a detoxification fast. These occur because your body reacts to the release of toxins from muscles and organs much the same way it would react to toxins released during a flu. Misinterpreting this "healing crisis" has caused many people to abandon a fast prematurely. Since these symptoms can be suppressed by simply starting to eat again, some people feel it is the right thing to do.

If you decide to detoxify by fasting, you need to realize that you are going to have bad breath, body odor, foul smelling urine and stools, and you're probably going to experience some aches and pains. When you consider that you're going to get rid of many of the poisons you've been carrying around for the last 20, 30 or even 40 years, it should be only a minor inconvenience to put up with. There are several things you can do that will minimize these problems.

1. **ENEMAS:** Your bowels are the main exit for toxic wastes during a fast. During a fast your bowels will most likely slow down and then probably stop. (Remember, if you are not eating anything, there's nothing to move through. Without an enema or some way of cleansing the colon, your body will reabsorb these toxins. The kidneys and lungs, etc., will help to eliminate some of the reabsorbed waste, but why overload them when a simple enema will do the trick?

    At least one enema a day is required and two is even better. A clear water enema (about 1 quart) both morning and night can cut down on the symptoms associated with fasting.

2. **EXERCISE:** Daily mild exercise like walking increases the circulation and the release of toxins. Your muscles act like pumps for your lymphatic system and help transport waste material from all parts of your body. Don't forget your lungs can also excrete more waste during exercise and deep breathing.

3. **BATHING:** Your skin is the largest organ of the body and it will eliminate between 1/4 to 1/3 of the impurities. Especially during a fast, a shower should be taken daily. Frequent brushing of the teeth and tongue scraping can also help.

4. **WATER:** Even if you're on a juice cleansing process. Make sure to use clean, pure water. Distilled water may be the best choice.

    If you have any kind of disease or are in poor health, don't attempt to fast without enlisting your doctor's advice and guidance. Remember also, fasting is a temporary means of detoxification and not a permanent means of eating.

5. **ELIMINATION DIETS:** There are several effective elimination diets that work to cleanse and detoxify the body without fasting. The 6 Day Elimination Diet is a good example of a very effective diet for this purpose.

THE 6 DAY ELIMINATION DIET

For six short days you will be on a FEAST, not a fast. You will be filling your body with nature's life-giving foods...fruits and vegetables that contain all those precious vitamins and minerals. When a sufficient amount of these live substances reach the cells of your body, there will be a flushing and cleansing such as you have never experienced before. You will eliminate toxic material that has been with you for years...toxic material that has robbed you of your vitality. After completing this diet, you will notice added energy, your complexion will undergo a marvelous transformation, you will sleep like a baby, aches and pains will seem to disappear and your nerves will be at ease. This is what the 6 Day Elimination

Diet can do. Follow the directions carefully and be sure that the quality of the fruits and vegetables that you purchase for this diet are of the highest available.

BREAKFAST:

Fifteen minutes before you are ready to eat breakfast, squeeze the juice of a lemon in a medium glass of hot water and drink it.

For each of the six days follow the breakfast menu below.

<u>Orange or Grapefruit Juice</u> - 8 oz. You can drink more, but be sure to drink at least 8 oz.

<u>Cottage Cheese</u> - 5 level tablespoons. (Due to the high beneficial bacterial content of cottage cheese and some soured milk products, there is usually no allergic reaction. However, be aware that this may vary from individual to individual and may need to be eliminated.)

<u>Fresh Fruit</u> - One-half pound. You may eat more, but be sure to eat at least one-half pound. Eat only one kind of fruit each day. (No bananas or avocados.)

<u>Herbal Tea</u> - No coffee or tea containing caffeine is allowed.

Between breakfast and lunch you should drink all the fruit and vegetable juice you can hold. Also, eat fresh raw vegetables and fresh fruit. The more live food you put down, the more thorough will be the cleansing. If you cannot get the fresh juices, then use the canned variety without sugar.

LUNCH FOR EACH OF THE SIX DAYS:

<u>V-8 Juice</u> - 8 oz.

Salad - Make a chopped salad of fresh raw vegetables. Use a dressing of olive oil, lemon juice and salt. Eat as much salad as you desire, but be sure to eat at least 8 tablespoonfuls.

Use four of the vegetables listed below for your salad:

Artichokes, Asparagus, Beans, Beets, Brussels Sprouts, Cabbage, Carrots, Cauliflower, Cucumbers, Celery, Dandelions, Endive, Eggplant, Fresh Corn, Fresh Green Pepper, Kale, Kohlrabi, Lettuce, Lotus, Okra, Onions, Parsley, Parsnips, Pumpkin, Radishes, Rutabagas, Salsify, Spinach, Squash, Swiss Chard, Tomatoes, Turnips.

Dessert - Fresh fruit with a little pure raw honey.

Herbal Tea

Between lunch and dinner drink all the fruit and vegetable juice you desire. Eat all the fresh fruit and vegetables you want.

REMEMBER...The purge comes from all the vitamins and minerals in the fruit and vegetables, so be sure to eat plenty.

DINNER FOR EACH OF THE SIX DAYS:

V-8 - Drink at least 8 oz., more if desired.

Cooked Vegetables - Select two or three of the different kinds listed under the salad section of the Lunch Menu. Steam them and season with a very small amount of butter if desired. Eat a generous helping of each vegetable. (No potatoes)

Bread - One medium slice of whole wheat with butter.

Dessert - Baked apple with cream or a salad of fresh fruit with a little honey.

<u>Herbal Tea</u>

If you feel hungry after dinner, eat fresh fruits and drink fruit or vegetable juice...ALL YOU WANT.

WHAT TO EXPECT FROM THE DIET:

The first day you may feel a slight discomfort by having changed your regular mode of eating, but do not allow this to disturb you for it is natural. About the third or fourth day, the bowels and kidneys will begin to move freely. Much toxic material will be passed. There will be symptoms of headache, perhaps nausea, gas, a few aches and pains, but do not become alarmed. About the fifth day you will feel a surge of energy. You will be surprised at yourself. Your complexion will have cleared up...your eyes will begin to brighten...you will feel wonderfully CLEAN inside. The little cells that were so full of toxins are now clean and they begin crying out for other food. Continue on until the end of the sixth day, then combine your meals as usual.

Note: If you start this diet, you must stick to it for the total six days in order to reap the benefits.

6.   **COLONICS:** Colonics are one of the most beneficial yet overlooked methods of detoxification. Basically, a colonic is a method of using water and oxygen to wash and clean the colon. It is much more efficient in cleansing than a simple enema and it requires someone with the proper equipment and training. A single colonic can sometimes do as much cleaning as a week of fasting or a three month cleansing diet.

Colonics used in conjunction with fasts can be responsible for some near miracles when it comes to correcting some chronic health problems, including allergies.

7. **SAUNAS:** Saunas are another method of detoxifying. Only use this tool if your doctor has determined you have a strong enough heart and cardiovascular system to handle the added workout it receives.

8. **CHLOROPHYLL:** Chlorophyll, the green juice from plants, has amazing abilities. It helps feed the beneficial bacteria in your colon, it neutralizes excess acid and helps remove and detoxify waste.

    Fortunately, there are now many excellent sources of chlorophyll including, alfalfa tablets, spirulina tablet or powder, wheat grass juice, barley greens or even liquid chlorophyll.

STEP BY STEP CELL AND TISSUE REPLACEMENT THE 7 YEAR SECRET

After detoxifying and removing wastes, you need to give careful consideration to what you put back into your body. What foods you eat will determine the quality of raw materials available for rebuilding and repair. In the case of allergies, or any ailment for that matter, you must consider all input to your body (food, water, air, environmental surroundings and attitude). Let's consider foods for example.

FOODS

If you know that you're allergic to certain foods, then avoid them initially. This may be necessary for several months. As your immune system rebuilds and improves, your abnormal reaction to certain foods will disappear. The time it takes will depend on several factors, such as: the efficiency of your detoxification, the severity and length of time you have had the allergy and how strict you are in implementing and maintaining a proper diet.

Total relief from food allergies can take longer than other allergies since your whole digestive system and immune system must be restructured and balanced.

Certain foods have a very high incidence of being associated with allergies. If you have allergies of any type avoid these foods initially also. These include, milk and dairy products, chocolate, sugar and shellfish. Let's look at each of these briefly.

A. Milk

Eliminating <u>milk and dairy products</u> from your diet may be the only thing you need to do to stop an allergy problem. For many people these foods never cause any problems, while for others, they are a perpetual source of misery. Why?

Milk contains two substances that can be difficult to break down...caseinogen and lactose. Caseinogen is one of the proteins of milk. The others are albumin and globulin. Even with the proper enzyme, caseinogen can be difficult to digest. Lactose can be even more of a problem. To breakdown lactose, you must produce the enzyme lactase. Lactase is normally produced to the age of 3 or 4 years and then production ceases. By this time, we no longer need it to digest mother's milk. In our society though, we still continue to ingest milk and our bodies usually adapt to this by continuing to produce lactose to around the age of 15 years. After that, production begins to decline or even stop in some people. If you continue to produce some lactose, you may be one of the ones that can consume unlimited milk and dairy products without much problem. Without lactose, these foods may contribute to allergies, sinus congestion, diarrhea, cramps, colitis, etc.

Heredity can also play a role in lactose intolerance. Blacks, Orientals and eastern European Jews have all shown a high incidence of being unable to handle lactose. Europeans seem to handle milk the best.

Some authorities even feel that milk may play an important role in aggravating other unrelated allergy symptoms even though you may not be bothered by milk itself. In other words, even if you don't demonstrate an allergic reaction to milk, by eliminating it from your diet, you may find that other substances you were "allergic to" are no longer a problem. Eliminate milk if you have a problem with allergies.

B. Sugar

Sugar has never been shown to be of any benefit to your health. Volumes have been written on the harmful effects of sugar. Sugar depletes numerous minerals and vitamins. It has detrimental effects on the pancreas, liver, adrenals, heart and bowels. It promotes tooth decay and promotes yeast infections by alkalizing the pH of the body. It aggravates a wide variety of ailments including allergies and arthritis. Sugar is not really a food, but only adds "empty" calories to the diet and contributes to the severe obesity problem we have today.

Any substance that depletes and stresses your immune system should be eliminated if you want to get rid of your allergies, and sugar is right at the top of the list.

C. Chocolate

Chocolate, besides being heavily laced with sugar, has some other bad attributes. Chocolate belongs to the same family as cocoa, cola, coffee and karay, a gum (vegetable gum). You probably know that all of these contain substances like methylxanthines and phenylethylamine that produce the "chocolate high". Do yourself a favor and eliminate the "foods" also.

D. Shellfish

Initially, you may need to eliminate shellfish also. Shellfish is very high in histamine. In fact, they contain a higher content of histamines than any other food. If you remember, histamines can cause the typical allergy symptoms: inflammation, swelling, and smooth muscle contractions. This is one food you may be able to reintroduce back into the diet after your digestive and immune systems are back in order.

Other common foods that you need to avoid initially, even though they should be a part of your diet later include: wheat and corn products, legumes, nuts, eggs and meat. If these foods cause no problems...don't eliminate them! Remember, the long range plan is not to eliminate and hide from foods that cause an allergic response. You may have to eliminate known problem foods in the beginning to keep from continually knocking down your immune system before it gets a chance to strengthen. Some foods you should eliminate forever, because they are simply detrimental to your health are sugar, fried foods, etc.

If you're not sure which foods you are reacting to abnormally, then you might try using the Pulse Test developed by Dr. Arthur Coca. It's not 100% reliable by any means, but if you find it works for you...then use it.

1. Take your pulse on the inside of your wrist when you first get up in the morning. (Remember, don't use your thumb to feel for your pulse...it has a pulse of its own.) Count the number of beats for one full minute. The average is between 60 and 80.

2. Now take your pulse again before you eat a single serving of the food you want to test. Only eat that one food. Take your pulse again in 30 minutes and then in 60 minutes after eating the food.

3. If you have an abnormal increase in the rate (10 points or more) this is supposed to indicate an allergy. (Remember that exercise, stress or an infection can also elevate your pulse.)

It would be impossible to list all of the allowable foods and all of the foods to avoid. Certain "foods" shouldn't be in anyone's diet whether they have allergy problems or not! You must continue to read and learn to properly adjust your diet. No one is perfect and everyone occasionally indulges in a "baddie" (strange we call them "goodies"...good for what?? Heart disease, diabetes, etc.). Moderation is the key. If you eat correctly 98% of the time your body can probably handle the other 2%.

Certain food groups should make up the majority of your diet.

Vegetables: Select a wide variety of vegetables. Different ones have different benefits to your overall health. Raw or steamed are the best methods of preparation. If you visit the local grocery store and can find over 3 or 4 vegetables you've never tried, you probably aren't getting enough variety. Eat vegetable dishes every day, not only for the many minerals, vitamins and chlorophyll they contain, but also for their excellent bulk. Don't forget the fresh salads with your meals too.

Soups: These are excellent foods that can be made with very little effort or expense. Eat soups regularly.

Whole Grains: Used as either cereals or in breads and pastas, whole grains should be used frequently. Brown rice, whole cracked wheat, rye, barley, corn and millet are excellent foods. As I mentioned, you may have to avoid corn and/or wheat for a short time.

Nuts: Nuts and nut butters are good, but only in moderation. Nuts are high in fat and may add unwanted calories. Cooking with nuts is one good way to enjoy their flavor without making them a total meal.

Beans: Rarely do they cause allergy problems; however, if not cooked properly, they may be difficult to digest. Beans could be included in your diet daily if you wish.

Seafood: As availability and prices improve, everyone should be able to include more seafood in the diet. Shellfish may need to be eliminated initially; however, deep-sea white meat fish a couple of times a week should be no problem. Cook by broiling and avoid prepared and battered fish cakes or sticks.

This is not an all-inclusive list, but only a small sampling of foods to include in the diet. It would be beyond the scope of this manual to cover all the permissible foods, recipes, etc.

Some Miscellaneous Tips On Eating, Choosing & Buying Food

*   Never go grocery shopping when you're hungry. You'll have a strong tendency to buy the wrong types of food. Your health and bank account will both be better off if you eat before you go to the grocery store.

*   Plan meals and make a grocery list that reflects the ingredients needed to make healthy meals. Stick to your list.

*   Give thanks either mentally or orally. Vegetables and/or animals have given up their existence to prolong yours. A long chain of people, from the farmer to grocery store clerks are partially responsible for your ability to have delicious wholesome foods.

*   If you have digestive problems, eat the heavier portions of the meal first.

    Meats are best digested at the beginning of the meal when hydrochloric acid in the stomach is

40

more abundant. Try eating the salads toward the end or throughout the meal.

* Chew all your food extremely well. Undigested protein molecules can cause irritation to the digestive tract.

DIGESTIVE ENZYMES AND HYDROCHLORIC ACID

Anybody with a food allergy probably has some digestive enzyme problems. It may not always be the answer, but many times an enzyme supplement can stop the body's abnormal allergic response.

Hydrochloric acid and various enzymes are necessary for the complete breakdown of foods into their smallest particles. Without proper digestion, large molecules of the undigested food are absorbed into the blood stream. These "foreign proteins" can evoke an allergic reaction.

A good combination enzyme formula usually will contain the following:

> betaine hydrochloride
> pepsin
> lipase
> pancreatin
> bile extract
> papain

It is best to take digestive aids following the meal. You still want your digestive system to produce as much hydrochloric acid and as many enzymes as it can before you interrupt the process. It is not uncommon to take several tablets (2 to 4) after each meal and gradually reduce the amount after a week or so. By gradually reducing the amount and watching for the return of the allergy symptoms, you can usually determine the proper amount needed.

There are several inexpensive tests that can be done by your doctor to check for hydrochloric acid and enzyme production. There are also a few obvious signs that may accompany a deficiency problem. If you have any of the following signs <u>and</u> an allergy problem, you may want to seriously consider adding a digestive aid complex to your program. All health food stores carry a variety of good digestive aid products.

1. Undigested food passing with bowel movements.

2. Excess belching, burping, bloating and gas after meals.

3. Constipation or low grade diarrhea.

4. Inability to digest minerals such as calcium.

5. If you are over 50 years of age (research has shown that at age 50 you are only producing about 15% of the hydrochloric acid you produced at age 25. Also, 35% of all individuals over 65 do not secrete any hydrochloric acid at all!).

THE ADRENAL CONNECTION

Since allergies are due to an abnormal response from your immune system, you must work toward strengthening and rebuilding it. The two areas of the immune system that generally need help when correcting allergy problems are the adrenal glands and the lymphatic system. Let's begin with the adrenals.

ADRENAL GLANDS

The adrenal glands are two small glands that sit directly above each kidney. They produce numerous hormones essential to life. A few of the actions performed by these hormones include:

*Regulation of blood sugar levels.

*Helping control blood pressure.

*Helping to provide resistance to stress.

*Fighting the blood vessel enlargement, swelling and fever associated with inflammation. Hormones produced by the adrenals are the body's natural anti-inflammatory compounds (cortisone).

*The adrenals also produce both male and female hormones in everyone regardless of sex.

A complete failure of the adrenal glands, called Addison's disease, fortunately is not common. If this does happen, hormone medication is necessary to preserve life. A more common occurrence is the condition hypoadrenia (low adrenals), where the glands are not quite capable of meeting all of the demands on them. After reviewing the many different jobs of these small glands, it's not too difficult to understand why a person with hypoadrenia can have a wide range of symptoms including: allergies, swelling in the ankles, feet and hands, fatigue, dizziness...especially on standing, weak knees, impotency, excessive urination, shakiness, depression, nervousness, chest pains, colitis and more.

Hypoadrenia is not normally found in standard laboratory testing; however, it is easily recognized by doctors familiar with the condition. A good history and general examination may be all that's necessary.

One of the screening procedures involves taking the blood pressure in 3 different positions and then checking for Ragland's sign. If you have a blood pressure cuff at home and know how to use it, you might try this yourself.

First, have someone record your blood pressure while lying on your back, then quickly sit upright and have it taken again. Then once more after standing. Normally with the help of your adrenal glands, your blood pressure will rise between 4 and 10 points (mm of Hg) going from the lying to standing position. If your blood pressure drops (the Ragland effect) it may be an indication of hypoadrenia. In fact, one of the common symptoms associated with hypoadrenia is getting a dizzy or "blackout" type sensation if you stand up too quickly.

If you have the condition called hypoglycemia (low blood sugar), you will almost always have hypoadrenia along with it. When blood sugar levels drop (usually from the roller coaster effect of eating refined sugar), the adrenals must work overtime by producing hormones that tell the liver to convert proteins to glucose in an effort to raise the blood sugar levels back to normal. Eating sweets depletes the adrenal glands.

Most diet and nutritional programs to correct hypoglycemia are actually geared toward strengthening the adrenals.

If you want to get rid of allergies, your adrenals must be in top shape. If you think about it, most allergy treatments involve the use of medications that are synthetic copies of the hormones produced naturally by the adrenal glands. All of the cortisone and anti-inflammatory drugs are an example. With a few simple procedures, you can rebuild and strengthen your adrenals so they can do their job. You can eliminate the need for the allergy shots and pills.

The adrenal glands have been nicknamed the "stress glands". To strengthen your adrenal glands you have to be familiar with the different types of stress and how the adrenals are involved.

In the 1920's and 1930's research by Dr. Hans Selye showed there are basically four types of stress and every one could have a dramatic effect on the immune system, particularly the adrenal glands. Let's look at each type.

1. MENTAL STRESS:

When most people talk about stress they are usually referring to mental stress. The death of a loved one, financial inability to pay bills, a dead-end job, or not being accepted by friends or loved ones are all good examples of the stress category. There are many methods of dealing with mental stress. Relaxation techniques, meditation, yoga, prayer, exercise and forgiveness are just a few. Everyone must discover their best method of dealing with mental stress.

A certain amount of mental stress is welcome and even beneficial for your mental and spiritual growth, but you must be able to control your reactions toward it and balance stressful activities with relaxation. If your occupation involves mostly mental work, then you can obtain a better balance in your life by relaxing with physical activities (exercise, woodworking, sewing, etc.). By the same token, if your occupation involves physically demanding activity, you can balance this with reading or other mental activities.

Oftentimes, you hear of the "fight or flight" mechanism when someone discusses stress. The classic example of "fight or flight" is the caveman walking through the jungle who comes face to face with a tiger. To survive, he has to either fight the tiger or run away.

Regardless of the choice he makes, his adrenal glands help him prepare for the "fight or flight". They increase blood pressure and heart rate to better circulate the new energy and oxygen carried to the blood, increase respiration for more oxygen and perform a host of other duties geared toward survival.

Whether the caveman fights or runs from the tiger, his activity would cause high levels of blood to be pumped through the adrenals and they would be replenished. The situation in modern times is different.

Even though you aren't confronted with life-threatening situations everyday, mentally stressful situations can cause the same response from the adrenals. Continued stress without allowing the adrenals to replenish their reserves can lead to a multitude of problems including allergies. You can give the adrenals a chance to replenish by working to control your reaction to mental stress and also by providing it specific nutritional requirements as you'll see later.

2. PHYSICAL STRESS:

Physical stress results from overworking, trying to do too much in one day and not giving your body adequate rest. Rest is just as important to the body as food and water. An organized routine that provides adequate rest balanced with sufficient exercise can do wonders for the adrenal glands.

3. CHEMICAL STRESS:

This type of stress is usually associated with pollution in our environment like pesticides, automobile emissions, etc. Although these are major components of chemical stress, usually our worst source is from our foods. Refined sugar, white flour, the thousands of preservatives, artificial flavors and colors being used, all place an enormous burden on your immune system and adrenals. Avoid refined sugars and white flour and start to minimize artificial and heavily preserved foods if you want to get rid of your allergies.

Prescriptions and over-the-counter medications are forms of chemical stress. These chemicals force the body to perform some action. You'll always have to pay more than just a monetary price for any benefits they bestow.

4. THERMAL STRESS:

Quick and drastic changes in temperature place an enormous burden on your body. Getting into an overheated automobile on a hot summer day and then immediately turning on the air-conditioner to blow on your face is excess thermal stress. Leaving a warm house improperly dressed for the winter cold is another example. It is best to avoid extreme changes in temperature.

Don't go overboard with this idea though. It's beneficial to experience seasonal temperature changes. Staying under a constant temperature with central heating and air-conditioning never lets your body fully adapt to the seasons. Your body operates on a biological clock and to be in harmony with your environment, it's necessary to experience the changes from night to day and the different seasons of the year.

Just as dietary changes (eliminating sugar, etc.) and exercise, nutritional supplements can also help replenish depleted adrenal glands. As you read through the recommended supplements, you'll probably notice that these are the same vitamins and minerals used to help allergy problems!

47

Vitamin C	From 2,000 to 5,000 mg
B-Complex	High potency (B-50 or B-100 type products)
Pantothenic Acid	250mg(Some authorities recommend as high as 2,000 mg/day for best results.)
B-6	50 mg

Adrenal glandular supplement

| Optional: | Vitamin E 400 IU
Vitamin A 10,000 IU |
| | Multi-vitamin and mineral complex with trace minerals |

(Publisher's note: Additional detailed information on both hypoglycemia and hypoadrenia solutions are available on a cassette tape program authored by Dr. Williams. Ask for cassette tape program #4 from Mountain Home Publishing, Box 829, Ingram, TX, 78025 (512) 367-4492. Cost is $6.00 postage paid.)

YOUR LYMPHATIC SYSTEM...MORE THAN JUST A 2ND SEWER

It's true, the lymphatic system works like a sophisticated sewer system, but it also makes up a large part of your immune system and can play a key role in allergy control.

The lymphatic system is an extensive network of tiny vessels and bean shaped structures called nodes. This network contains twice the amount of vessels as the circulatory system and has two times the amount of fluid as your body has blood. Its jobs are many.

The lymphatic system returns fluids that leak from our bloodstream. As blood circulates through arteries then capillaries and then into veins, it leaks certain fluids. These fluids must be returned to the blood stream, but first they are filtered through lymph nodes. Specialized lymph nodes are the main filters of your bloodstream.

They also work to neutralize toxins and infectious material. Foreign materials can enter the lymph system many ways, but our diet plays the major role. Improper dietary habits place an extra burden on the kidneys and liver forcing them to cleanse the impurities in the blood. This constant overload of fats, toxins and mucus eventually spill over into your lymphatic system. This extra burden can impair its ability to perform its immunity chores.

Your lymphatic system produces white blood cells and antibodies. When you "back-up" or overload your sewage system, everything is affected. At one time or another, you've probably felt a congested lymph node in the neck, armpit or groin. Congested, hard working nodes, are swollen and tender to touch. Their discovery can be quite alarming especially if you suddenly find the mysterious lump and have no idea what caused it or where it came from.

Congestion in the lymph system is not uncommon. It has a more difficult time than our circulatory system moving fluid because it doesn't have a heart for a pump. Lymph fluid is moved by breathing, walking, intestinal activity and muscle action. As muscles tighten, lymph vessels are squeezed and lymph fluid is pushed along through the system on its way back to veins that lead to your heart. Much like your veins, lymph vessels have small valves to keep the fluid from traveling in the wrong direction. Your thymus gland, tonsils and spleen are also a part of the lymphatic system.

A stagnant or overloaded lymph system can lead to the production of abnormal antibodies which trigger allergic reactions. Fortunately, there are several easy ways to improve and help the lymphatic system.

A. Proper diet is essential. Excessive fats, sugars or mucus forming foods like milk and dairy products can clog even the most efficient system.

B. Improving your bowel habits lowers any extra work on the system. Constipation dumps an enormous load of toxins and wastes back into the blood stream. Initially the liver and kidneys may be able to handle this, but eventually the lymphatic system becomes involved.

C. Dehydration can cause a sluggish congested lymph system. Make sure you are drinking a minimum of 8 glasses of water daily.

D. Exercise is necessary. A rhythmic contraction of your muscles will efficiently pump the waste material and fluids thru this filtering system.

Exercise isn't just for the heart and lungs. Your entire body thrives on movement and activity. In a somewhat indirect way, a good walking program can help your allergies as well as strengthen your heart.

E. Massage benefits the lymph system. Just remember to always massage in the direction of the heart. Trained massage therapists realize that massaging in this direction increases lymphatic drainage and improves the overall health of their client. For someone who is absolutely too weak or debilitated to exercise, this may very well be the most effective method of helping them regain their health.

F. A slantboard used for ten to fifteen minutes twice a day is another easy way to help. You may have to start out staying only five minutes the first few days and gradually increase the time. (* If you have a serious medical problem, consult with your doctor before using a slantboard. Certain conditions can be made worse. Don't use a slantboard if you have high blood pressure, pelvic area cancer, hemorrhages, tuberculosis, ulcers, appendicitis, etc.)

G. Vitamin C and A have been found to help lymphatic flow.

H. Nutritional glandular supplements of the thymus and /or spleen may also help in lymphatic congestion. Thymus glandular supplements used by children with persistent tonsillitis have shown to be highly successful.

I. Even light exercise on a "bouncer" helps. A bouncer is a device made up of a heavy duty woven mat attached by springs to a metal frame (similar to a small version of a trampoline). Almost anyone can use one with great success. As you bounce up, your muscles work against gravity and as you come down, fluids such as lymph are helped to move upward to your heart.

THE NERVOUS SYSTEM

Not all allergies are related to the reaction between an antigen and an antibody. An imbalance of your autonomic nervous system (ANS) can result in an abnormal response by your body.

An example of this would be where a particular food triggers muscle contractions in the intestinal tract. Asthma, hay fever and hives can sometimes fall into this category. You may have even read or heard of people who are allergic to heat and cold. These are classic cases of someone with an unbalanced autonomic nervous system (ANS). If you are like most people, you're probably asking: "Just what is this autonomic nervous system and what does it have to do with allergies?"

The ANS is the portion of your nervous system that controls the glands, those found in the bowels and urinary tract. This division of the nervous system is closely related to the adrenal glands and can be influenced by some of the same things. Sugar, drugs, animal fats and stress can make your nervous system over-sensitive. Over sensitivity in a person has been described as being a "bundle of nerves". The nervous system over-reacts to stimulus that would otherwise cause no problem. I have literally seen people's hands swell from holding a cold object when the ANS is out of balance.

All of the methods I described earlier to strengthen the adrenal glands will also help balance your ANS; however, there are other areas you need to consider if you think this is a problem.

The vertebra or small bones that make up the spine can become misaligned (subluxated) and cause nerve irritations. Lifting, falls, bad sleeping positions, automobile accidents or hereditary weaknesses can all lead to misaligned vertebra (subluxations). In cases such as this, corrections to the spine should be performed by a competent doctor of chiropractic.

Sometimes acupuncture can help balance the ANS. Your nervous system is a complex electro-magnetic and chemical communications system and many things in the environment can throw it out of balance. Fluorescent lighting and microwave radiation are just a couple of examples. Some of the most unusual cases have been helped through a balancing of the acupuncture circuits.

OUTLOOK, ATTITUDE AND ALLERGIES

Every thought and emotion influences the hormonal and nervous systems, which in turn can influence the body's immune response. Mental outlook and attitudes can play a major role in allergy control.

Some researchers feel emotions can influence allergies because of the "placebo-effect". A placebo is an inactive substance which doesn't produce any direct activity by the body. Placebos, in one form or another, have been shown to give relief or cure in thousands of different conditions (including allergies) between 30% to 50% of the time. Just by placing complete faith and trust in a particular therapy, pill, etc., you can tremendously influence your health.

Many allergy therapists now incorporate some type of "behavior modification" program such as yoga, dance, biofeedback or visualization into the treatment. These types of therapies are far more effective placebos since you are actually calling on your inner resources to help in the healing process. The real cure or healing is always done by the body. We can only make sure it has the proper raw materials it needs. We can accomplish this by a proper diet, exercise and mental attitude.

In dealing with allergies you must adopt the attitude that allergies are simply an indication that your body is not in harmony with the environment. You are not fighting a war against hostile plants or cat fur. An allergy can be a wonderful opportunity to strengthen your entire structure. Remember, there is no war against allergens, there is no enemy. The problem again is simply a matter of not being in balance with your surroundings.

CHAPTER 7

GUIDELINES FOR CHANGE

The ideas in this chapter don't really fall under any one topic that has been covered; however, they need to be included. You should find these guidelines helpful in eliminating allergies and most all illnesses you encounter.

1. Just as you should expose yourself to and experience the different seasons, you should also expose yourself to different stimuli. Learn and listen to the opinions and viewpoints of others. Isolating yourself from people you disagree with is similar to hiding from allergens. You don't have to accept or agree with everyone. Those with whom you disagree are no enemies, but just part of your environment that can serve to strengthen your own ideas while still helping you remain flexible to adapt to change.

2. Bathe everyday. The massaging action to the skin is healthful and bathing creates a sense of freshness and vitality.

3. Eat slowly and give your body time to digest properly.

4. Maintain active communication with your family members. Let them know how thankful you are that they are part of your life.

5. Enjoy the outdoors everyday if the weather and your health permits it. Just a few minutes a day spent outdoors can have long term effects on your mental well-being.

6. Make sure you have some "quiet time" to yourself everyday. Life passes fast enough without going through weeks or even months not reflecting on who you are as an individual and giving thanks to everyone who has given you support and guidance along the way.

7. Live each day without dwelling on sickness. A change from sickness to health or from depression to happiness rarely occurs overnight. More than likely you will have both, good and bad days with the good ones becoming more frequent as your health improves. Expect and visualize health.

8. If you have difficult phases. It helps to read about or talk to others who have experienced similar circumstances. Don't forget those who are now experiencing what you have in the past. Your support could be of great benefit to both of you.

9. Marvel at nature and the process of creation. Realize that your ability to change and the ability to make decisions about your life are two of the most wonderful gifts you have to use while here on Earth.

CHAPTER 8

NATURAL ALLERGY REMEDIES...TEMPORARY HELP FOR SPECIFIC PROBLEMS

Everybody wants quick relief from allergies and the quicker the better. Because of this, I have compiled several remedies that have helped many through their suffering. Keep in mind that these are not cures for allergies. Until the digestive and immune systems are brought back into balance, you will only be treating a symptom of the problem and not the cause.

By using these various remedies in conjunction with the information in the rest of the manual, you can gain temporary relief while working on a permanent solution.

HAY FEVER AND SINUSITIS

This is one of the most common forms of allergy. Medically, it is referred to as allergic rhinitis. It involves both, an allergic response and an inflammation of the nose. The typical symptoms are concentrated in the head: runny nose, watery eyes, sometimes fever, stuffy head, ear pressure and sneezing. The nose feels as if someone has used sandpaper to clean it due to the irritations of constant blowing and removing the constant clear watery discharge.

The allergic response can be too many different types of pollen. Common ones are from trees, grasses or weeds. Molds can also cause problems.

NUTRITIONAL SOLUTIONS

Vitamin C

2,000 mg to 5,000 mg spread throughout the day (400 mg to 1,000 mg every 3 hrs. for example)

If you're using ascorbic acid as your Vitamin C source, be sure to take at least 500 mg of calcium daily. High doses of ascorbic acid can cause a loss of calcium. To avoid any calcium loss, use calcium ascorbate for your source of vitamin C.

Bioflavanoids

500 mg to 1,500 mg daily (These should be spread throughout the day and they must be taken at the same time as vitamin C to be effective.

	Additional bioflavanoids can be taken in the form of grated orange or lemon peels mixed with a small amount of raw honey. One teaspoon twice a day has often worked wonders by itself. If you have trouble sleeping because of hay fever, try 1 teaspoon of this mixture 10 minutes before bedtime.)
B-Complex	1 tablet daily of a supplement that contains 50mg of each B vitamin (Many products are labeled B-50, etc.)
Pantothenic Acid (B3)	200 mg to 500 mg daily

Optional Supplements to Enhance the Above:

Digestive Enzyme Complex	1 or 2 tablets 10 minutes after each meal
Vitamin E	200 IU to 500 IU daily.
Evening Primrose Oil	
EPA Fish Oils	Preliminary studies have shown it may help in some asthma cases.

A combination of the following supplements have been used by several doctors and reported to be quite effective:

Niacin	50 mg to 100 mg three times a day (With niacin, be aware of the flushing sensation that may occur.)
Tyrosine	This is an amino acid and can be found in any health food store.
Pyridoxine (B6)	100 mg to 250 mg daily

ADDITIONAL RECOMMENDATIONS AND THERAPIES

1. Quit Smoking!

2. In persistent problems, you may have a sinus infection. In these cases, flushing and cleaning the sinus cavities is beneficial. Purchase a nasal inhaler bottle and fill it with a solution called D.A.G. It is a solution of phenolated iodine in an Irish moss extract with organic borates (iodine, sea weed and sea water). D.A.G. can be found in most health food stores or from the distributor:

Sun Country, USA
P. O. Box 15524
Phoenix, AZ 85060
In Arizona (800) 532-7487
Outside Arizona (800) 528-3613

This solution can be used several times throughout the day as needed. It is not a medication and doesn't cause the "rebound effect" I mentioned earlier. Make sure you get the solution back into the sinus cavities when you inhale. It may cause a burning sensation which is considered normal.

3. In persistent sinus problems the possibility of an infected tooth should be ruled out by your dentist. Many people have suffered for years only to later learn that a chronic tooth infection was the culprit.

4. Reflex points located just on either side of the nostrils can sometimes promote sinus drainage. Firm fingertip pressure applied to these points in a rotating circular motion for 30 to 45 seconds is suggested.

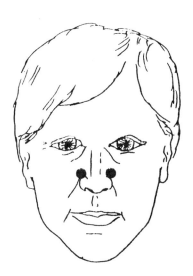

5. The use of local raw honey can be used to acclimate your immune system to pollens in a certain locale. It must be raw and uncooked. It

may not help immediately, but if 1 or 2 teaspoons are used daily for 6 months to a year, the results are usually very worthwhile. Honey works on the same basic principle as desensitization shots without the expense or discomfort.

6. Several herbal teas help break-up and remove mucus. These include Fenugreek, Slippery Elm and Flax seed. Fenugreek tea seems to work best on thick mucus or mucus deep into the chest.

7. Allowing the sinuses to drain can sometimes bring relief. Since the sinus cavities are open only on the top, you can lie on your back and let your head hang off the side of the bed to help drain them.

8. DMSO can be used effectively on sinusitis caused by allergies. First, a 70%-90% solution can be applied topically on the skin directly over the sinuses. Secondly, a 30%-50% solution can be applied with a cotton swab directly to the internal nasal passages themselves. This latter method may be painful for the first few minutes due to the greater sensitivity of the mucous membranes.

    Both of these methods have shown to be very effective since DMSO has the ability to reduce inflammation. It is not uncommon to have large amounts of and quick relief from the pressure-type headaches accompanying sinusitis.

9. Water-soluble chlorophyll, either in capsules or liquid can be diluted with water and sprayed into the sinuses. Since the chlorophyll complex has a tendency to break down, it is best that the solution be freshly made about every two days. This is a very inexpensive method that works well. Chlorophyll is readily available at all

health food stores. All that's needed is about 2 or 3 capsules or 1 teaspoon of the liquid mixed with enough water to fill the small spray bottle.

10.   The above spray can be alternated daily with a solution of two teaspoons of apple cider vinegar to one pint of distilled water. This solution helps balance the pH of the mucous membranes.

ASTHMA

Asthma involves an abnormal response involving the constricture of the bronchial tubes leading to the lungs. You may have asthma with or without allergies. Asthma has been described as trying to breathe while a car is parked on your chest. Almost 10 million Americans suffer from asthma. It is the most common chronic disease of children and will probably remain so, as long as children are fed high amounts of sugar and foods high in artificial coloring and preservatives.

Asthma is one condition you may be able to blame on your mother, which I'm sure she'll be happy to hear. Next time you talk to her, ask her if she felt depressed, worn-out and fatigued during the first five or six months of the pregnancy and then experienced an enormous boost of energy and vitality during the last couple of months. Sometimes after giving birth, the mother also feels extremely depressed and fatigued again. If this happened and you now have allergies, asthma, hypoadrenia or hypoglycemia, she may be partially the blame.

If the mother starts the pregnancy with an uncontrolled hypoglycemia (low blood sugar) or hypoadrenic condition, the extra stress will only further deplete her adrenals for the first several months. However, later in the pregnancy, the baby's adrenal glands develop and begin to function. Since their circulatory system is connected, the mother can begin to use the baby's adrenals; hence the burst of newfound energy. This continues until the baby's birth. The mother feels like the "rug has been jerked from underneath her" and the baby is left with a weakened immune system, weak adrenals and probably hypoglycemia.

There are several helpful temporary solutions to asthma, but true permanent relief requires an intense program of strengthening the immune system.

NUTRITIONAL SOLUTIONS

(The same nutritional supplements recommended for hay fever and sinusitis should be used in asthma cases. Be sure to support the adrenals nutritionally also.)

ADDITIONAL RECOMMENDATIONS AND THERAPIES

1. Electronic air filters that can be placed in the central heating and air conditioner ducts are a great help while indoors. Small table air filters that use foam or woven mesh filters are not nearly as effective.

2. Humidifiers can help in dry climates or during winter months when heated indoor air loses its moisture content. *Be especially careful to regularly clean all humidifiers and filter screens. Their damp surface provides an excellent breeding ground for mold and spores which can be circulated throughout the house. Many people have traced their allergy problems to an uncleaned humidifier or filter element.

Check all household appliances that have circulation or cooling fans for heavy dust or mildew buildup. One common appliance that may be blowing allergens all over the house is the refrigerator. Be sure to thoroughly clean the coils there.

3.   I mentioned that you could have asthma with or without allergies. Asthma is one of the conditions that can be a result of a nervous system imbalance. Since the constriction of the bronchial tubes is under the control of the nervous system and uninterrupted, undisturbed nerve supply to this area is essential.

I have seen more cases of asthma controlled or corrected through chiropractic adjustments than by any other means. This form of treatment shouldn't be included under temporary forms of relief since a nervous system imbalance can be corrected through chiropractic treatment. If this is the primary cause of the asthma, you can obtain permanent relief. Adjustments to the neck and upper back areas can sometimes even stop an asthma attack in progress.

SKIN ALLERGIES

Hives, eczema and a host of other skin conditions fall under this category. These two in particular, have been linked to certain foods such as eggs, shellfish, fruits and nuts. Eliminating the few items would be simple enough, but food is not the only thing blamed. Medication, sunlight, exercise, pollens, chemicals, insects, etc. have also been listed as causes.

It's easy to see why doctors have such a difficult and unsuccessful time treating skin allergies. Practically everything has been implemented as the cause. Creams, lotions and medications are applied to the skin while the patient takes other drugs orally, all in an effort to stop what the skin is made to do...eliminate toxins.

All skin diseases (including allergies) are not simply a problem with the skin itself. All skin diseases have one thing in common...they are an indication of a build-up of toxins or waste materials in the body. Your skin is not just a covering stretched over a bony frame to protect your internal organs. The skin is your body's largest elimination organ and it is a reflection of what's going on internally.

When other elimination and detoxifying organs become overloaded or unable to function properly, the skin begins to help. Weak liver function has been related to psoriasis. Adrenal insufficiency and excess refined sugar in the diet contributes to seborrheic dermatitis. Skin disease can be traced to a malfunctioning intestinal tract, kidney or liver dysfunction, a clogged lymphatic system, weak adrenal glands or even an unbalanced thyroid. I have discussed several of these areas in the manual and suggest you re-read those sections if you have a skin disease or allergy. I haven't said much about the kidneys, liver or thyroid glands, so just briefly let's take a look at their role in skin disease.

The kidneys are one of the organs used to filter and cleanse the blood. Any detoxification program can help the kidneys by reducing their workload. Also, certain foods such as milk and milk products, sugar, chemicals and drugs (especially antibiotics) tend to weaken them. A low water intake can keep them from flushing the concentrated waste they hold. Weakened kidneys along with the liver can be an underlying cause of skin disease.

An overworked liver can result in psoriasis and other skin problems. Sugar, food additives and chemicals can and do weaken the liver, but the over consumption of meat, especially pork severely limits its detoxifying ability. Eliminating all sugar and pork products from your diet along with supplements to strengthen the liver can help even the worst cases of psoriasis.

The thyroid controls the functions of three layers of skin. Problems with this gland are often overlooked when it should be one of the first areas to check in skin disease cases. A hypo-thyroid condition can cause hair loss, extremely dry skin, cracked hardened heels and a long list of skin diseases. If you suspect a thyroid condition, a simple inexpensive check can be made using a thermometer.

THYROID CHECK

1.   You need to make sure your metabolic rate is normal and the easiest way to do this is by taking your temperature.

Remember:

* Shake the thermometer down before retiring.

* Upon awakening, place it in your armpit and leave it there for at least 10 minutes before getting out of bed.

* Record the temperature below.

Note: Men can take their temperature anytime. Women in their menstrual years get the most accurate reading on the 2nd or 3rd day after menstrual flow starts. Before the first menstrual period or after menopause, the temperature can be taken on any day.

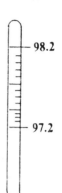

98.2

97.2

Anywhere between these two temperatures (97.8 to 98.2) is considered normal. If you are outside this range, see special note below.

YOUR TEMPERATURE IS_____

SPECIAL NOTE

Anything below 97.8 usually indicates a sluggish or hypo-thyroid condition.

Publisher's note: A special cassette tape program by Dr. Williams outlining the natural methods of balancing the thyroid is available from Mountain Home Publishing, P. O. Box 829, Ingram, TX 78025. Total cost $6 postage paid.

Skin diseases pose a double problem. First, they are influenced by internal toxins and waste. Secondly, when these toxins are released through the pores they can react with substances you come in contact with. This form of allergy, contact dermatitis, can make it difficult to touch anything from money to cosmetics. Rather than spend a lifetime avoiding contact with every possible allergen, time needs to be spent cleansing and detoxifying. When the protective oils and fluids released by your skin are contaminated with toxic waste, no cream, lotion or medication will ever be the answer.

ADDITIONAL RECOMMENDATIONS

1.   Temporary relief of inflamed skin can sometimes be achieved with common household ingredients.

*   Ice or ice packs applied directly to the site of the inflammation for 10 to 15 minutes can help stop the itch and pain. A simple effective ice pack can be made by blending ice cubes with a small amount of water for a short time in a blender. Then wrap this "ice slush" mixture in a cotton dish towel and apply it to the area of irritation.

*   A mixture of 1/2 water and 1/2 vinegar will many times help soothe an irritated area.

*   Warm (not hot) baths can offer relief from many skin conditions. Many authorities recommend adding skim milk powder, cornstarch, baking soda or even a small amount of bleach to the bath water.

*   In addition to products found in the home, either calamine lotion or zinc oxide paste from your local pharmacy may be applied to most skin allergies.

2.   Try to use natural fabrics such as cotton for your clothing and bedding materials.

3.   Avoid dry cleaning if possible.

4.   Have your doctor check any medications you are taking for possible allergic side effects. Even many of the prescribed and over-the-counter creams and salves recommended for skin allergies can themselves, trigger reactions.

5.   If you must handle cleaning solvents or irritating liquids around the house, wear heavy rubber coated gloves at the time. These

"weather proofed" or "liquid proofed" gloves are available at most hardware stores and will provide better protection than the so-called rubber gloves sold to protect your hands from dish water.

* These are only a few precautions you may need to take initially with contact dermatitis and skin allergies. The following additional information may help in determining what substance or substances you may be reacting to abnormally.

ARTIFICIAL COLORINGS:

These colorings or dyes are processed from coal and may or may not be specifically listed on a label. Butter, cheese and ice cream, for example, need not list any artificial colors used in their ingredients.

Blue No.1   Red No.3
Blue No.2   Red No. 40
Citrus Red No.2   Yellow No.5
Green No.3   Yellow No.6
Orange B

ARTIFICIAL FLAVORS:

BHT and BHA:

These preservatives are used widely to preserve oils and foods high in oil such as nuts, cereals and fried snack foods.

Caffeine:

This occurs naturally in coffee, tea and cocoa and is commonly added to soft drinks.

Calcium Propionate:

Inhibits mold formation.

Caramel Color:

Used to deepen color and made from heating various types of sugars.

Casein:

The same protein in milk that is added to cause thickening in a product.

Citric Acid:

Known as vitamin C and occurs naturally in many foods, but is added to some. Can cause sensitivity reactions in some people.

Food Starch:

Usually derived from corn, wheat, arrowroot, tapioca or potatoes.

Malt:

Yeasted-fermented corn, wheat or barley is its source.

Monosodium Glutamate (MSG):

A flavor enhancer derived from soybeans, corn, wheat, sugar beets or seaweed. Commonly found in oriental foods and responsible for headaches sometimes associated with "Chinese Restaurant Syndrome".

Gums:

Rarely a problem, but bothersome. Derived from various sources including : carob, guar, ghatti, carrageen, chicle, karaya, tragacanth and arabic.

Potassium Iodine:

Added to salt.

Sodium Nitrite:

Used in pork, fish and luncheon meats as a preservative.

Sulphur Dioxide:

Prevents discoloration and bacteria growth.

Sweeteners:

These are numerous and frequently used in all types of food products. They include: aspartame, corn syrup, cyclamate, dextrose, glucose, mannitol, saccharin, sorbitol and sucrose (table sugar).

AUTOIMMUNE DISEASE

An abnormal response to the environment is the most common form of allergy; however, increasingly we are seeing diseases in which the body abnormally reacts towards its own tissues.

Normally, the body is able to differentiate its own cells from those foreign to it. When this ability is lost, it can attack and destroy its own tissue, causing irreversible damage throughout the body. The "autoimmune" disease includes: multiple sclerosis, pancreatitis, certain anemias, rheumatoid arthritis, hepatitis, some kidney diseases and possibly adult onset of diabetes.

Even though some authorities feel that autoimmune diseases are caused totally by either a virus or strain of bacteria, further study shows that not everyone exposed to a specific bacteria or virus will actually develop the disease. In fact, the disease may never manifest or only come to light when the immune system weakens.

This is a prime example of where an inherited weakness or tendency to develop a disease may be overcome by maintaining a strong immune system.

Just about anyone who suffers from rheumatoid arthritis knows how certain foods can aggravate the problem. The offending foods are usually stimulants like soft drinks, coffee, sugar, chocolate or honey which weaken the immune system further by depleting the adrenal glands. An improper diet can turn a minor arthritic into a cripple.

Even with all the evidence relating to diet, constipation, stress, mental attitude, etc. to the development and progression of autoimmune diseases, almost all treatment programs avoid dealing with these areas completely. The therapies of choice today, lean toward massive doses of drugs like cortisone, surgical removal of immune organs like the spleen or blood transfusions. All of these are used in hope of weakening the immune system's response (normal or abnormal).

While possibly affording some temporary relief, they greatly increase the chance of developing other serious diseases down the road. Pausing for just a few minutes to study the overall picture should convince even the most cynical that intentionally weakening the body's immune system can't be compatible with long term health.

Whether you presently have an autoimmune disease or not, you should be leery of drugs, excess alcohol, radiation, hormones like estrogen and even some mega-vitamin therapies. All of these have the potential of weakening the immune system and may either induce or exaggerate an autoimmune disease.

Also, a wide variety of chemical irritants present in the water and the environment now have the ability to mutate and damage normal body cells. The "mutated" or foreign cells may then trigger an allergic response causing the formation of antibodies capable of destroying normal cells and tissue.

In addition to all of these, new generations of drugs and therapies are currently being developed that can alter or influence our genetic code and our DNA molecules. God only knows what type of autoimmune diseases we'll see in the future.

RECOMMENDATIONS

If you presently have an autoimmune disease, every effort possible should be made to strengthen your immune system. This type of disease is an unmistakable sign that a breakdown of the immune system has occurred! The road of recovery must start with a thorough detoxification and cleansing program followed by the most natural wholesome diet possible and careful attention to proper attitudes and emotions.

Autoimmune diseases are not incurable. In fact, the breakdown of the immune system is a highly unusual occurrence. Your immune system has the natural ability to restore and maintain health and when it has the proper support it will do just that. Health is the normal, not disease.

In addition to the nutritional suggestions for strengthening the adrenals, etc. mentioned elsewhere in this manual, a few other supplements have been found to help in autoimmune diseases.

1. Trace minerals, such as zinc, selenium, lithium and the mineral iron are particularly important in these conditions.

2. Vitamin E has been shown to stimulate and help strengthen the immune system in several studies. Amounts as high as 1,600 IU a day have been recommended.

3. Vitamin A can help the thymus gland and overall immune system, but excessive amounts may be toxic and even aggravate certain conditions. (Authorities usually recommend between 10,000 IU and 25,000 IU daily.)

4. Proper digestive enzymes are essential. Other natural enzymes found in foods like bromelain (in raw pineapple) and papain (in papaya) help break down proteins as well as help the formation of immune system cells.

5. Certain amino acids such as cysteine, arginine and ornithine may also help.

6. High dosages of vitamin C have been shown to block or stabilize many of the symptoms of autoimmune diseases. In severe cases, the daily amount is usually determined by "bowel tolerance". The daily intake is that amount that almost, but doesn't quite cause diarrhea.

CHAPTER 9

YOU MAY NOT HAVE AN ALLERGY...YOU MAY BE POISONING YOURSELF!

An allergy is an abnormal reaction to a substance that is normally harmless to others. Allergy-like symptoms; however, can also be a normal response to some chemical irritant or poison. Although this is not a complete list by any means, here are a few of the common ways you may be slowly poisoning yourself without realizing it.

1.   Humidifiers and filter systems can be prime breeding areas for unusual and sometimes dangerous molds. Legionnaires disease has been traced to similar problems in air-conditioning cooling towers. Either white vinegar or borax in warm water is an effective solution for removing molds.

2.   Radon gas is an odorless, tasteless, radioactive gas that is naturally formed in nature by the breakdown of uranium. It is responsible for between 5,000 and 20,000 cases of lung cancer each year. It can seep into homes built over uranium rich soils. Certain areas in

Pennsylvania, New York and New Jersey have been shown to have exceedingly dangerous levels in many residential areas. For more information on testing and the dangers of radon, I would highly recommend obtaining two free consumer guides. <u>A CITIZENS GUIDE TO RADON</u>, OPA-86-004 and <u>RADON REDUCTION METHODS</u>, OPA-86-005 can be obtained by sending a postcard to Environmental Research Information, 25 West St. Clair Street, Cincinnati, OH 45268. From the same source you can also request a free manual called <u>RADON RADIATION TECHNIQUES FOR DETACHED HOMES</u> (EPA 625/5-86/019), which details for contractors and home owners, who have the tools and skills, ways to reduce radon concentrations in the home.

3. The fumes given off by natural or propane cooking and heating appliances can cause serious problems, especially in homes that are well-insulated or have inadequate ventilation.

   Burning natural gas gives off carbon monoxide, nitric oxide, formaldehyde, nitrogen oxide, benzene, acetylene and other gases. This happens not just during cooking, but continuously if you have a pilot light burning. If you notice your allergy symptoms (headaches, stuffy or runny nose, etc.) go away when you're out of the house, you should consider switching to electricity. If this isn't possible, improve the ventilation especially during cooking and turn off the pilot light.

4. Some air fresheners (aerosol and solid) give off a cancer-causing chemical called paradichlorobenzene. Use baking soda instead to absorb odors.

5. Check for asbestos and urea-formaldehyde foam insulation in older trailer homes and buildings.

   Formaldehyde test kits are available from various sources or you can contact your local state board of health who may test your home for free. Although asbestos and urea-formaldehyde have recently been banned, new building materials (particle board, new carpeting, etc.) still contain formaldehyde. Once these materials age and "gas out" there is usually no problem, but you may need to neutralize the gas initially.

   To neutralize formaldehyde, place a bucket in each room containing 1 tablespoon of ammonia in one gallon of water. Close the house and leave for several hours. When you return, open the windows and doors to air out the house and remove the buckets. Ammonia chemically inactivates the formaldehyde. If necessary, you may do this every few months until the building materials sufficiently age.

6. Check for and minimize your exposure to pesticides and cleaning solvents around your home and place of work.

7. A polluted or tainted water source can cause serious problems. Living in the country with your own well doesn't always insure a clean water supply. Runoff from heavy pesticide use is now reaching most underground and surface water supplies. If your water supply is suspect, consider buying or making distilled water.

CHAPTER 10

SOURCES OF NATURAL PRODUCTS AND SERVICES

Publisher's note:

The listing of products and services that follow are not endorsements as such by the author or publisher. They have been beneficial sources for many allergy sufferers as well as those wanting to use "natural" products in their homes and businesses. We encourage you to investigate each source by reading the labels and contacting the manufacturers directly about specific ingredients or production methods in question.

AIR FILTERS & PURIFIERS:

Allergen-Proof Encasing, Inc.
1450 E. 363rd St.
Eastlake, OH   44094
Phone: (800) 321-1096
          (216) 946-6700

Mail order: (Vitaire HEPA air filters)

Bio-Tech Systems
P. O. Box 25380
Chicago, IL 60625
Phone: (800) 621-5545
              (312) 465-8020

Mail order: (Cleanaire HEPA room air filters, Tech Dust Guard furnace filters)

BEDDING

The Cotton Place
P. O. Box 59721
Dallas, TX 75229

Mail order: (100% cotton blankets, sheets, pillowcases, towels, pillows, etc.)

Feathered Friends
155 Western Ave. West
Seattle, WA 98119
Phone: (800) 426-2724
              (206) 282-5673

Mail order: (Down comforters and pillows with 100% cotton products, also will recover old down comforters)

Scope Natural Fibers
3576 Stacy Circle
Lumberton, NC 28358
Phone: (919) 738-8897

Mail order: (mattresses of natural cotton)

CARPETING:

Dellinger, Inc.
P. O. Drawer 273
Rome, GA   30161
Phone: (404) 291-7402
Mail order: (carpeting without dyes or other finishes
and 100% cotton carpeting)

CLEANING SUPPLIES:

Bio-Tech Systems
P. O. Box 25380
Chicago, IL   60625
Phone: (800) 621-5545
              (312) 465-8020

Mail order: (mold preventative spray)

Bon Ami Company
1025 W. 8th Street
Kansas City, MO   64101
Phone: (816) 842-1230

products available in most retail grocery stores (Bon
Ami non-chlorinated soap and powders, without
perfumes, dyes or ammonia, also polishing cleansers
and glass cleaners)

I. Rokeach & Sons, Inc.
560 Sylvan Ave.
Englewood Cliffs, NJ   07632
Phone: (201) 568-7550

products available in most retail stores (Rokeach
kitchen soap which is made with coconut oil)

COSMETICS:

Caswell-Massey Co., Ltd.
518 Lexington Ave. at 48th St.
New York, NY   10017
Phone: (212) 755-2254

Mail order: (cosmetics and skin care without dyes,
synthetic materials or perfume)

The Community Soap Factory
P. O. Box 32057
Washington, DC   20007
Phone: (202) 347-0186

Mail order: (pure coconut oil, natural soaps, soaps
made without animal products)

GK Laboratories
Londonderry, VT   05148
Phone: (800) 451-4453
            (800) 824-3103

Mail order: (petroleum jelly without the petroleum,
made with pure lanolin and olive oil)

Salonique
P. O. Box 1959
Fort Worth, TX   76101

Available through professional hair care salons
(hypoallergenic hair care products)

FOODS

Elam's
2625 Gardner Road
Broadview, IL   60153
Phone: (312) 865-1612

Mail order: (grains, flours, mixes, cereals and peanut butter)
Ener-G Foods, Inc.
6901 Fox Ave. South
Seattle, WA   98124
Phone: (206) 767-6660

Mail order: (gluten free, wheat free pasta, mixes, flours, baked goods and brans, milk powders and substitutes.)

Kennedy's Natural Foods
1051 W. Broad Street
Falls Church, VA   22046
Phone: (703) 533-8484

Mail order: (Their catalog is designed specifically for people with food allergies and people on restricted diets. Products include: breads, cakes, canned goods, carob products, cereals, condiments, dried fruits, nuts, milk substitutes, flours, grains, herb teas, jams, jellies, oils, pastas, etc.)

Olde Fashioned Foods, Inc.
123 N. 18th Street
Fort Smith, AR   72901
Phone: (501) 782-6183

Mail order: (honey, fruits and vegetables, flours, cheeses, meat, poultry, teas)

FORMALDEHYDE SEALER:

Mortell Co.
Dept. HC
550 N. Hobble Ave.
Kankakee, IL   60901

available in retail outlets: (Hyde-chek formaldehyde
vapor barrier)

NUTRITIONAL SUPPLEMENTS:

Allergy Research Group
2336 C. Stanwell Circle
Concord, CA   94520
Phone: (415) 685-1228

Mail order: (supplements without preservatives,
fillers, binders, colors or lubricants, also have a
Vitamin C derived from sago palm rather than corn)

Willner Chemists, Inc.
330 Lexington Ave.
New York, NY   10157
Phone: (212) 685-2538

Mail order: (nutritional supplements without artificial
coloring, sugar, starch, etc.)

PEST CONTROL

Allergen-Proof Encasing, Inc.
1450 E. 363rd St.
Eastlake, OH   44094
Phone: (800) 321-1096

Mail order: (insecticide spray for night and day)

Homesteader's Warehouse
P. O. Box 2330,Dept. 6287
Roseburg, OR   97470

Mail order: (natural odor traps for garbage flies,
yellow jackets and fruit flies)

PET CARE:

Westward's Herb Products Co.
P. O. Box 1032
Studio City, CA   91604
(213) 761-1112

Mail order: (shampoo, powders, conditioner, etc. made
from herbal sources)

EPPCO
3350 Ulmerton Rd. Suite 8
Clearwater, FL   33520
Phone: (813) 577-5643

Mail order: (herbal shampoos, powders, etc.)

WATER DISTILLERS:

Water Wise, Inc.
26200 Hwy. 27 South
Leesburg, FL   32748
Phone: (800) 874-9028
              (800) 321-5141 (in Florida)

Retail: (Dol-Fyn Water Distiller)

BIBLIOGRAPHY

Abrahamson, E.M., and Pezet, A.W., <u>Body, Mind, and Sugar.</u> New York: Avon, 1951.

Aihara, Herman, <u>Acid and Alkaline,</u> Oroville, CA; George Ohsawa Macrobiotic Foundation, 1980.

Ballantine, Rudolph, M.D., <u>Diet & Nutrition, A Holistic Approach</u>, Penn.; The Himalayan Institute, 1978.

Billman, Alice. <u>Guidelines for Ecological Living.</u> 1982. Available from: Human Ecology Research Foundation of the Southwest, 12110 Webbs Chapel, Suite 305 E, Dallas, TX 75234.

Blanchard, Edward B., and Epstein, Leonard H., <u>A Biofeedback Primer,</u> Reading, MA: Addison-Wesley, 1978.

Bricklin, A.S., <u>"Natural Healing, The Ultimate: How the Body Defends and Repairs Itself"</u>; in the Practical Encyclopedia of Natural Healing, Bricklin, M. (ed.), pp. 179-185, 332-359, Emmaus, PA; Rodale Press, 1976.

Brown, Barbara B. <u>New Mind, New Body.</u> New York: Harper & Row, 1974.

Coffin, Lewis, <u>The Grandmother Conspiracy Exposed.</u> Santa Barbara, CA: Capra Press, 1974.

Crook, William G., <u>Are You Allergic?</u> Jackson, TN; Professional Books, 1974.

Dickey, Lawrence, Ed. <u>Clinical Ecology.</u> Springfield, IL. Charles C. Thomas, 1970.

<u>Dietary Goals For the United States,</u> Washington, D.C.; National Academy of Sciences, 1982.

<u>Diet, Nutrition and Cancer</u>, Washington, D.C.; National Academy of Sciences, 1982.

Dufty, William, <u>Sugar Blues</u>, New York; Warner, 1975.

Forman, Robert. <u>How to Control Your Allergies</u>. New York; Larchmont Books, 1979.

Fredericks, Carlton, and Goodman, Herman. <u>Low Blood Sugar and You.</u> New York; Grosset & Dunlap, 1969.

Faelten, Sharon and Editors of Prevention Magazine. <u>The Allergy Self-Help Book,</u> Emmaus, PA. Rodale Press, 1983.

Gerrard, John W., <u>Food Allergy: New Perspectives.</u> Springfield, IL; Charles C. Thomas, 1980.

Giannini, AV, Sculz, N.D., Chang, T.T., Wong, D.C., <u>The Best Guide to Allergies,</u> New York; Appleton-Century-Crofts, 1981.

Golos, Natalie, and Golbitz, Frances. <u>Coping With Your Allergies.</u> New York: Simon & Shuster, 1978.

Kushi, Michio, <u>A Natural Approach to Allergies</u>, Tokyo and New York; Japan Publications, 1985.

Kushi, Michio, <u>Diabetes and Hypoglycemia,</u> Tokyo; Japan Publications, 1985.

Mackarness, Richard. <u>Chemical Victims</u>, London; Pan Books, 1980.

Mendelsohn, Robert S., M.D., <u>Confessions of a Medical Heretic</u>, Chicago, IL: Contemporary Books, 1979.

Miller, Saul, M.D., <u>Food For Thought,</u> Englewood Cliffs, NJ; Prentice-Hall, 1979.

Pfeiffer, Guy O., <u>The Household Environment and Chronic Illness</u>. Springfield, IL.: Charles C. Thomas, 1980.

Randolph, Theron & Moss, Ralph. <u>An Alternative Approach to Allergies</u>. New York: Harper & Row, 1980.

Stevens, Laura J., <u>The Complete Book of Allergy Control,</u> New York: MacMillan Publishing, 1983.

Truss, C. Orian, <u>The Missing Diagnosis.</u> 1983. Available from: P. O. Box 26508, Birmingham, AL 35226.

William, Roger J., <u>Nutrition Against Disease</u>. New York: Pitman Publishing, 1971.

Zamm, Alfred and Gannon, Robert. <u>Why Your House May Endanger Your Health.</u> New York: Simon & Shuster, 1980.

INDEX

Spirulina 34
Steroid-type drugs 4
Stress 13
Sugar 37, 66
Sulphur Dioxide 72
Sun Country, USA 60
Sweeteners 72

T
Thermal stress 47
Thymus gland 75
Thymus glandular supplements
    51
Thyroid check 67
Thyroid glands 66
Tonsillitis 51
Tooth decay 37
Tyramine 21
Tyrosine 60

U
Ulcers 8

V
Vegetables 39
Vision 8
Visual disturbances 7
Vitamin A 48, 75
Vitamin C 12, 13, 48, 51, 58, 75
Vitamin C complex 12
Vitamin E 12, 48, 59, 75
Vitamin K 12
Vitamin therapy 15
Vitamins 15, 30, 37, 39, 47
Vomiting 8

W
Water 30

Wheat grass 34
Whole Grains 39

Y
Yeast infections 37

Z
Zinc 74